Urban Goddess Mama

How I Got My Goddess Back After Postpartum Depression

Melania Tolan

Melania Tolan
PO BOX 16222
PORTLAND, OR 97216
www.urbangoddessrevealed.blogspot.com

Publisher's Note: The author acknowledges the copyrighted or trademarked status and the trademark owners of any workmarks mentioned in this work of nonfiction.
The author does not dispense medical advice. Please consult your medical provider for treatment and advice.

Cover Design by Christy Caughie at http://gildedheartdesign.com

Photo by Eric Hudson

Book Layout © 2014 BookDesignTemplates.com

Urban Goddess Mama/ Melania Tolan. -- 1st ed.
ISBN 978-0990400707

To All the Goddess Mamas in this World

CONTENTS

Dearest Reader,

Thank you so much for purchasing my book. If you are a new mom or mom-to-be, congratulations and I shower you with love and blessings. You are in for a wild ride. Along the way you'll have some unforgettable experiences you will cherish forever and challenging ones that will make you cringe. Enjoy it all. Every day will bring something new and, no matter how bad it gets, bedtime does eventually come, followed by a new day. If you are a new father or father-to-be, kudos to you, too. Your role as a new parent is going to be equally challenging as you learn to nurture both your child and partner. Whether you bought this book because someone close to you is dealing with "baby blues" or just to learn more about postpartum depression, I applaud your interest in an issue that affects a great number of women after childbirth. According to BabyBluesConnection.org, 80 percent of new mothers experience baby blues and 1 of 5 new moms is diagnosed with postpartum depression.

When I started to write *Urban Goddess Mama*, it was primarily a way to process what happened and what went wrong after the birth of my child—basically my own personal therapy. But when I got to the 10,000-word mark, I realized this wasn't a story to keep to myself. As I dealt with the debilitating effects of postpartum depression, I realized thousands of women suffer from this disorder, many of whom never seek treatment or support because of the stigma and shame associated with the diagnosis. Why is it you can talk about getting cancer or a cold and no one bats an eyelash, but the second you mention depression or any kind of psychological disorder, suddenly you become the white elephant in the room?

After months of shame and fear, I decided no more. My goal in writing and publishing this book is to provide an insider's view of what it is like to experience, treat, and move past postpartum depression. Postpartum depression is real, and it can have irrevocable consequences if left untreated. The good news is that there is help out there and lots of hope.

My deepest desire is that you will find this book helpful. If there is one thing you can take from my story to make your life better, I have accomplished my mission. Thanks again and let's start the journey together, shall we?

Much love,

Melania

CHAPTER ONE

New Beginnings

Let me start from the beginning and give you a little background on my life. At age 33, I had everything going my way. I had a new career with the opportunity to work from home, a budding writing career by night, a fabulous husband who loved me exactly the way I was, and a cozy home in the city of Portland. I was surrounded by fantastic family and friends. All of these things made me feel like maybe I was ready to start a family.

I'd always been healthy. I exercised, kept a relaxed vegetarian diet, and made sure I got my eight hours of sleep every night. My spiritual life was thriving as I had joined a wonderful group of women years before who inspired me to add magic and beauty every single day. I meditated and prayed. Yoga was my best friend. I spent time outdoors, something not hard to do in the beautiful Pacific Northwest.

So when I decided to get pregnant, I envisioned myself as the all-natural, crunchy-granola, earth mama: bathed in glowing light, wearing flowing natural fiber clothing, my infant close to my breast in a Moby wrap as I strolled through the farmers' market filling my fair-trade basket with organic vegetables and herbs. Grace would become my middle name, and everyone I encountered would be blessed by my radiance. Oh yes! I was full of delusions of grandeur.

But that is where the fairytale ends and the true story begins. It was the Friday before Memorial Day 2012.

All week I'd been eating like a proper little piggy. One day I actually went to the cafeteria at work five times and bought full meals. This was in addition to filling my plate at the department potluck because I was so hungry. One of my coworkers teased, "You're pregnant. Ha ha."

Ha ha indeed.

That Friday I woke up at three a.m., my coworker's words echoing in my ears. Oh boy, what if she was right? I remembered I had a pregnancy test stuffed under the bathroom sink and practically jumped out of bed with anticipation. For the first time in my life of peeing on the "stick," it came out positive. I sucked in my breath as the plus sign filled the tiny window. *Here we go.*

I'd always known that when the time came to have a baby, I'd want a natural birth (obviously) either at home or at a birthing center. I'd watched *The Business of Being Born* and knew I was a healthy person who wouldn't need to be in the hospital.

When I found out I was pregnant, it seemed natural for me to pick a midwife and birthing center. I went with a local midwifery center, which came highly recommended by a personal friend and other acquaintances. Over the nine months of pregnancy, I received top-notch care from the nurse practitioner midwife and her two assistants. My only hang-up was that none of these women had children, but I squashed that feeling and didn't say anything because I liked them very much.

I was happy and reassured when my ultrasounds and labs throughout the pregnancy were normal. This validated the decision to have my baby at the birthing center rather than the hospital.

I had one appointment at the beginning of my pregnancy with the obstetrics office I used just to make sure everything would be okay. They also did all my ultrasounds. Originally I was supposed to see Dr. B, but the appointment had to be rescheduled because of an emergency procedure she was called away to perform.

I was bummed because I really liked her. She treated her patients well, and, being a mother herself, she understood what they went through. Instead I saw her partner, Dr. D. He'd delivered many of my friends' babies and operated on some of them, too. I trusted him and his opinion, and he reassured me everything looked fine with me and Baby.

Later that year in December, my husband and I took a *Birthing From Within* childbirth class, and we really enjoyed it. I discovered I could cope with pain well, as we had to hold ice in our hands while practicing the breathing techniques taught in class. I even bought the book that the class was based on and found it insightful. The art exercises were particularly helpful in dealing with the anxiety leading up to the actually birth. Yet I couldn't quite shrug the feeling something was missing or that I didn't feel very prepared. I kept telling myself these emotions were normal for new moms.

In my head, I had this vision of myself laboring in a luxurious tub filled with warm water at the birth center while my midwife coached me through the birth. I'd swum throughout most of the pregnancy and even wrote a mermaid young-adult novel over the summer so it only seemed appropriate that my daughter would be born in the water. Yeah, I was going to be the ultimate Zen water goddess mama, surrounded by candlelight and tranquility as I brought my little princess into the world.

The last trimester flew by like a torpedo, as we were busy with the holidays and getting everything ready for Baby to come the first week in February. My pelvis had been hurting badly, and I'd been going to see the chiropractor regularly for adjustment. However, the treatment on Friday, January 18, didn't seem to do much good, which worried me a bit.

My midwife was gone for a long weekend, but I wasn't concerned because this was my first baby and firstborns always come late. The next day, Saturday, I had my last prenatal massage. On Sunday, Hubby and I attended an infant CPR and first aid class.

Before the class, I went for a nice, relaxing swim. I swam longer than usual, and felt great. On the way home, I stopped by the store and bought some last minute items—just in case. That night, I finished up a book review for my blog, completed some other projects, and a few chores.

At three in the morning on Monday, I turned in bed and felt like I was going to pee my pants. I rushed to the bathroom, just in time to feel the gush of water pouring out of me, and it wasn't my bladder at work.

My first thought: "Oh shit, my midwife is out of town." My second thought: "Is it okay to text the assistants at three in the morning to tell them my water broke?" I don't want to be rude, you know.

My husband, who normally works nights, happened to be home this particular morning and encouraged me to call them, which I did.

One of the assistants called me back. She told me to stay home and to check in with them when the contractions started and expect one of them to come over in a couple of hours. I texted my boss and told her I'd be working from home. She was very understanding. I worked for four hours, mainly wrapping up loose ends just in case this was my last shift before maternity leave.

Hubby finally installed the car seat that my folks had bought us and had been sitting in the living room for two months.

Around nine in the morning, the assistant came over and checked me. She said it could take hours before my labor began but suggested I rest and take it easy. I took the remainder of the day off and laid down for a nap next to my husband, who had gone back to sleep to be rested when the time came.

About an hour later, I woke up and realized my contractions had started. They felt like severe menstrual cramps, similar to those I experienced battling endometriosis in my early twenties. I thought, "This isn't too bad. I can handle this." The contractions became more regular and within the hour they started coming every five to seven minutes. Each one grew in intensity to the point I couldn't lay in bed anymore.

I got up and started doing some last minute stuff around the house—finishing packing my birthing center bag and throwing in some laundry—anything to mask the anxiety that came with each contraction.

As my contractions increased in intensity, all sorts of thoughts danced in my head, making me dizzy. What if I can't do this? What if I die? Worse, what if the baby dies? Oh, god, I'm going to end up in the hospital! I texted the midwife assistant and told her what was happening, minus the hurricane of fear brewing inside my gut. I didn't want to appear weak. She came over again.

When she knocked on my door, I was having a contraction leaning on the yoga ball, and couldn't even move to open it for her. That's how intense they were. Honestly, I don't know what early labor is because I went into active labor so quickly. Within minutes, the pain became unbearable. I got in the shower on my hand and knees. The hot water hitting my back seemed to take the edge off and let me breathe through the contractions. Water, blessed water. If I had water, I knew I could do this.

Soon afterward, the assistant came in and said it was time to go to the birthing center. Yes! That meant I was close. However, on the way there as we were pulling off the freeway, I had this crazy thought that I should tell Hubby to turn right instead of left and take me to the hospital. A strong contraction kept me from saying anything other than, "Oh hell, this hurts."

We arrived in the early afternoon. As soon as the tub was filled, I got in and relaxed into my labor. *Water goddess, here I come.* I let the water hold me, felt its warm embrace as I concentrated on opening my body to let the long-awaited child through. This is what I'd been waiting for. Unfortunately, it didn't last long.

I became cold as the water cooled. We added more hot, only to realize it was cold. Somehow they had run out of hot water for that particular room and tub. *Oh no, this couldn't be happening.*

To make matters worse, the room was cold, too. I shivered as I got out, which only made the contractions worse. By this point I couldn't take the pain. I became very vocal with each one. *Holy shit, it really did hurt.*

"Lower your voice," one of the assistants said, "and send that energy to your baby."

What? How does one send energy to a baby? I thought. *Furthermore, why would I want to send this pain to the baby?* She repeated this several times and told me to say "open" during the contractions. I did, but it didn't help with the pain or reduce the intensity. This was *not* the serene, natural, earthy childbirth I had anticipated. The longer it went, the deeper my fear festered.

At some point, the substitute midwife came in and introduced herself. She seemed pretty nice, but we didn't connect at all, mostly because I was in utter agony. To me, she felt like another assistant but not involved. Most of the time she stood in the shadows, letting the assistants do all the work and occasionally asked them how I was doing. She checked me after a while and said I was almost dilated and could start pushing soon.

By now it was dark outside, the fireplace was lit, the light turned down low, and candles burned everywhere. I looked around the room and thought this was the environment I wanted, but now that the time had arrived, none of it helped soothe my raging emotions. Boy was I ready to have this baby. I'd had enough of the pain. Baby needed to come and the sooner the better.

I pushed for what seemed like an eternity, but it was more like an hour or so. When the midwife checked me, I was fully dilated, but the baby hadn't moved down the birth canal. She suggested I walk around. I laughed. I could barely move; it hurt so much. The drugs at the hospital started to sound more appealing with each contraction.

For most of this, I didn't even know where my husband was. Turns out he'd left the room because he couldn't handle me screaming in pain and no one doing anything to ease it. That's what he told me later. He wanted to help so badly but didn't know how.

For natural pain relief they finally suggested I bounce on a yoga ball in the shower. And so I did. There I was, in a tiny slate-tiled shower stall, on the ball. Hot water cascading down my body, warm steam enveloping me; I was in my element at last. I drew strength from each droplet. The heat eased my pain, and I entered labor-land alone but fully empowered.

I felt like a goddess on her throne, finally able to focus my energy on pushing and opening rather than the pain of childbirth. Those forty-five magical minutes were exactly how I had envisioned my labor would be.

Unfortunately, when I came out of the shower and the midwife checked me, she said the baby still hadn't dropped. The baby also needed to turn her body and head slightly so she could move down the birth canal easier. Without the warm water therapy, the pain returned with a vengeance. The assistants tried different techniques to get the baby to turn, but the only thing that happened was more pain.

At this point I realized it could be hours before Baby came, and I had run out of steam. I was tired and had had enough. I remember thinking the whole natural birth thing was bullshit and pain-relieving drugs sounded really good. The epidural at the hospital called my name and I answered.

As requested, Hubby loaded me up in the car, and, with the accompaniment of the assistants, I was whisked to the hospital. I wept during the drive to the hospital, knowing this wasn't what I wanted but what I needed now. Yet a little voice whispered, "You should have listened to me when I suggested you turn right instead of left earlier. It would have saved you so much pain and suffering."

Within minutes of arrival, the anesthesiologist came in and administered an epidural. It took another ten minutes before I started feeling the effects. Relief! That doctor was the hero of the night, as far as I was concerned. If my legs hadn't been numb, I would have crawled out of my hospital bed and kissed him right then and there.

Now that I was at the hospital, my care was transferred to the midwives on duty at the hospital. The moment I met the night-shift midwife, I knew I should have been here the whole time. Every cell of my body knew this because I felt the tension melt away in that second. Between the labor nurses and the midwife, I knew I was in the presence of women who'd traveled down the road through birth-land. They understood my pain. The comfort this brought gave me hope that maybe I could get through the night and possibly actually have this baby.

They let me sleep for three hours. Blessed rest, finally. Oh, how my body and mind needed it. About three in the morning, the midwife started me on Pitocin, a labor-inducing medication. She started with a miniscule amount, measuring the pressure of my contractions with a catheter inserted into my uterus and adjusting the dosage accordingly. I had control of how much epidural medicine I received. This made me feel less guilty about my last-minute decision for medical interventions.

I was pretty numb but still could feel the pressure with each contraction. This allowed me to breathe through and focus on relaxing my pelvic muscles—a much better way to labor after the ordeal from the previous day. By eleven in the morning, it was time to push again.

To my amazement, they had me pushing in all sorts of positions. Hands and knees on the bed while the nurse and midwives held my knees and legs steady. Squatting at the foot of the bed, holding onto a bar. A whole variety of positions. I did not expect this from a hospital birth. In the hospital births I'd witnessed, the woman was strapped to the bed with her feet up in stirrups. That was the main reason I didn't want a hospital birth in the first place, but now I questioned all my decisions.

Had I made a mistake in going with an independent midwifery clinic rather than choosing the hospital midwifes? Doubt moved in. If I couldn't choose the right care that I needed, how would I be able to make decisions for the child I had yet to birth? Thankfully, I didn't have time to dwell on these things as all my focus fixed on pushing. *Please come out, Baby!*

After two hours of pushing, the midwife said the baby was stuck behind the pelvic bone. More than twenty-four hours had passed since my water broke, and she was concerned about the risk of infection, especially since I had had a urinary tract infection before going into the labor. She called in the surgeon to discuss my options. After everything I'd gone through, the thought of surgery freaked me out. He offered me a choice between vacuum and forceps or C-section. I wanted to avoid the latter at all costs so I chose the vacuum. He explained that while there were risks, because the baby had descended so low and just needed a little help turning her head and coming under the pelvic bone, she was a good candidate for this option.

The room filled with medical staff: three NICU nursing team members to resuscitate Baby in case she stopped breathing; my nurse; the midwife; the two midwife assistants from the birthing center; the baby's nurse; the surgeon; his assistant; and Hubby. Talk about a birthing "party." There I lay on the bed, propped up by pillows in all my naked glory, but I didn't give a rat's ass about modesty.

The only thing I cared about now was getting Baby out because I was tired. If I didn't do it now, the scary "C" loomed over me like a haggard witch with long, grubby fingers waiting to snatch my baby girl from me. I could almost hear her cackles. By golly, I wasn't going let her win after all my hard work. At least not if there was a chance I could still deliver vaginally.

Ready, set, go! Let's do this thing. I started to push again on the doctor's cue. With each push, he suctioned the baby's head down a little more. On each contraction, he coached me on where to push and for how long. I didn't think I had any more strength left, but the doctor encouraged me and somehow I found a few extra ounces of hidden energy. Like an angel sent from the heavenly realms, he guided me through the last leg of my wild birthing journey. Four contractions and my baby girl came out.

When I saw the slimy, bloody, little human lying in his hands between my legs, my heart almost stopped.

I'd spent most of my life not wanting kids. Sure, I loved children—other people's offspring, that is—but I'd never felt the urge to procreate myself. I had spent my entire adult life avoiding getting pregnant. I also didn't think I would ever marry either. I was pretty happy living my own life. Then I met my husband. Everything changed. I knew I could be a wife to him and bear his children within the first week we met. For someone independent like me, that said something about the awesomeness of the man who's my partner, best friend, soul mate, lover, and spouse. And now we finally had our daughter.

The nurse put my baby on my chest. I held her close and kissed her wet, gooey, little head of black hair. She was mine. All mine. I'd done it. I'd carried her for nine months, felt her kicks, talked to her, wondered what she'd look like, and now she was here in my arms. They took her away for a few moments to do her assessments and vitals but brought her right back. Skin to skin, she lay on my chest. One slow wiggle at a time, she made her way to my breast. Within twenty minutes she found my left nipple and latched on naturally.

While I bonded with my daughter—which was more like "let the shock sink in" that I was a mother now—the surgeon sewed up my perineum. I had a third-degree tear. I didn't feel it because of the epidural. I didn't care, though, because I'd avoided a C-section and I had Baby vaginally. I owed that man a debt of gratitude for helping me bring my little angel into the world, even if she did have a cone-head thing going on from the vacuum extraction.

Once the drugs wore off, I did care about my condition. I couldn't sit, much less walk, because of the stitches and my bruised tail bone. The baby's head had done a number on my pelvic area. It felt like someone had taken a bat and machete down there. Oh, my! And trying to pee was like spraying acid on a raw wound.

I questioned what the hell I had been thinking, and, in my dark state of mind, I wondered if a C-section might have been a better option. *Who thinks that?* I mentally slapped myself. For once, I understood why some women chose that route, and I knew I would never ever judge them. It hurt just to pass gas, and I freaked out about when the time came to poop. The midwife put me on stool softeners which helped. Ice packs and good ol' narcotics helped ease the discomfort.

Oh, and did I mention sore nipples? Yes, breastfeeding is amazing and great for bonding and the baby's health, but OH. MY. GOD. OUCH!!! Yet it didn't matter to me because I was determined to breastfeed my daughter even though my nipples felt on fire every time she nursed.

Unfortunately, breastfeeding did not come easy. I had lactation specialists come in every day during my hospital stay, sometimes several times during the day, showing me how to get Baby to latch on and encouraging me to pump after every feeding. So not only was I waking up every two hours to feed her, I had to spend another fifteen minutes pumping a few extra drops of colostrum and then clean the equipment so it would be ready for the next use. It felt pointless to try to sleep in between feedings.

Shortly after I delivered, I spiked a fever. The midwife put me and the baby on antibiotics. I wanted to cry every time I looked at the clean diaper wrapped around her right arm to protect the IV line. The invisible words written all over the white material flashed at me: "You did this because you chose to come to the hospital. Because you were too weak to have her naturally."

The second day at the hospital, Baby became jaundiced. She spent twelve hours under bilirubin lights—the longest day ever while we were in the hospital. The sight of the machine next to my hospital bed was just another slap in the face for my failure.

The third day, when we should have been going home, our blood work revealed I was fine but my daughter's white blood cell count had gone up. The good news was that her immune system worked; the bad news was that we needed to stay for another two days so she could complete her antibiotic regime, even though her blood cultures came back negative. The pediatrician said it was better to keep her two more days than to go home and risk having her become ill. A second hospitalization would be worse. I completely agreed.

We were transferred to the Children's Hospital next door. It felt silly having NICU nurses taking care of my baby just to have antibiotics administered when other babies were there with much more serious problems. At least they had one easy patient.

The following day, her IV became infiltrated and a new one had to be put in. Hubby had gone home to get a few things, and I didn't have the courage to watch the procedure alone. The medical staff took her into another room. The whole time, I felt like the worst mother for not having the strength to be there for my baby, but I simply couldn't watch unless they were ready to put an IV in me and give me a sedative. A half hour later, the nurse told me they are going to get the IV specialist. Another half hour passed. The nurse said they couldn't get the IV in, and they were calling the care flight nurse because she was the best. Well, she couldn't do it either. Finally they talked to the doctor to see what other options were available for administering the antibiotics. It turned out she only needed three intramuscular shots and that was it.

The nurse felt awful, but I felt worse when I saw all of the Band-Aids covering Baby's body. If I learned anything from the experience, it was that my little girl is one tough cookie and stubborn as a bull, kind of like her mama used to be. If only I had been stubborn enough to birth her at the center and avoid all of this.

The next morning her blood test showed everything was normal, and we were allowed to go home. Bringing home Baby was the best gift imaginable. We received the highest-rated care possible in the hospital. All of the nurses, midwives, lactation specialist, and doctors rocked. But there was nothing like being home. Little did I know the hardest part hadn't even begun.

CHAPTER TWO

Black Fog

I was so relieved to come home. The first twenty-four hours felt like heaven, not having well-meaning nurses coming in to check on me and Baby every two hours. But by the second day, I started to break down. My little girl was crying something fierce. I sat on the yoga ball with her in my arms, bouncing up and down for what seemed like eternity. The stitches down there didn't help matters. Hubby sat in a nearby chair, resting before his turn to bounce Baby.

I remember turning to him and saying, "It's a fucking miracle the human race has survived this long because this right here sucks ass." I loved my child, but I hated that moment.

He nodded in agreement. Eventually the baby did go to sleep, and we were able to go to bed and get some much-needed rest. Two hours later we started from square one again.

By the third day home, my milk finally came in strong. Hurrah! I felt relieved I could finally feed my baby and not supplement with breast milk a girlfriend had generously donated. However, my appetite had not returned. In fact, food was a real turn off. My mother had come to visit the day we got home and brought us food and fresh juices for me. The fridge overflowed with food, but none of it looked or sounded good. Not even my favorite comfort foods like mac and cheese or mashed potatoes enticed me. Nothing appealed to my palate, but I needed to eat to maintain my milk. All of my friends wanted to bring me food, but that was the last thing I wanted. Even though I didn't have an appetite, I still got hungry. Standing in front of the fridge, starving but with nothing appealing to me has to be one of the worst forms of torture possible.

The only thing I could tolerate was cold cereal, but it had to be unsweetened and have as little flavor as possible. Plain oatmeal, corn mush, and multigrain unsweetened granola with almond milk became my staple one or two times a day. I forced myself to snack on Wheat Thins and unsalted raw pecans. It wasn't much, but at least I was taking in calories and it wasn't junk food.

A few days after we came home, Hubby had a ticket to see the band Muse play at a local arena. One of my favorite groups, I'd been looking forward to seeing them, hoping Baby would come a few days late so I could go to the concert. My sweet husband knew this and told me to go.

"What?" I gasped. "And leave my baby so soon?"

"She'll be fine. We have milk here from our friend so if I need to feed her I'm set. Go, you deserve this." He practically pushed me out the door.

I'd never gone to a rock concert alone, and the last thing I wanted was to be around thousands of people—I couldn't even handle close friends and family at this point. My husband's coworkers were there, but I didn't know them well so I felt like I was alone, surrounded by an overwhelming amount of people.

When Muse came onto the stage, everything I was dealing with or had gone through up to that point melted away. For two hours, I forgot about all of my issues and the fact I was sleep deprived. For two whole blessed hours, I was transported away. But even as I enjoyed the music, I realized how much my life had changed and sadness overwhelmed my brief respite of joy. It hurt to dance, and I had to sit most of the time during the show, although sitting wasn't very comfortable either. Tears of guilt stung my eyes. I should be at home taking care of Baby. What mother leaves her newborn to go to a rock concert?

Nothing was about me anymore. I had to put my baby girl first. I mourned the loss of my independence but felt selfish thinking those thoughts. I should be happy, swooning over my little angel, but what I felt inside was the opposite. I almost resented her, and the shame for feeling that way overpowered every other emotion.

The bills started to arrive shortly after I came home from the hospital. I needed to add Baby to my insurance since I had better coverage than Hubby's policy provided. But that required me to fax or drop off the paper work to Human Resources. Since I didn't have a fax machine, dropping them off was my only option—just another thing to do to the growing list. By adding her to my insurance, I would have an extra $2,000 deductible to worry about. The combined medical expenses pretty much ate our allotted savings for maternity leave. I'd lay awake at night while the baby slept soundly, wondering how the hell we were going to pay for everything. I worried I might need to go back to work before the end of my maternity leave—a prospect I did not look forward to.

Days and nights melded together to form a murky vortex where time flowed by, but I couldn't tell you from where it came or went. Every two hours I nursed, burped, and changed Baby. She would then fall asleep on me, and I would be stuck sitting in my recliner most of the day. It was as if she was attached to my chest 24/7. The hours flew by. One moment it was morning then it was seven o'clock at night. I couldn't tell you what day it was or what hour. Most of the time, I sat in my recliner with the baby on my chest, staring off into space, unaware of what played on the TV or where Hubby was in the house. Basically, lights on but no one home. My mind clouded with a fog so dark everything I looked at or thought about appeared black.

Two weeks after the delivery, Baby developed thrush and generously transferred the yeast infection to my nipples. Not only were they sore, but now they burned with a pins-and-needles pain radiating deep into my breasts. At the same time, my vagina started to itch like mad, but I couldn't bear to touch the area because I was so sore.

Pain in the ass (literally), itching crotch, hunger with a lack of appetite, burning nipples, pumping milk after every feeding, screaming baby, lack of sleep, fluxing hormones, stressing about finances, and never a moment to myself—it was the perfect recipe for postpartum depression. Did I mention the tears? Yes, I cried all the time and at the littlest things.

At my two-week postpartum appointment with the birthing center midwife, the stress escalated. The midwife assistant took the baby to have her weighed. She weighed seven pounds, nine ounces. When she returned, she said I wasn't giving my daughter enough milk because she should have returned to her birth weight (seven pounds, thirteen ounces) by two weeks. Great. So I wasn't properly feeding my baby after all. My heart sank. Tears welled up in my eyes. *Don't cry. Do not cry*, I told myself over and over again. Crying would show weakness and God forbid they witness that, too. It was bad enough I hadn't been strong enough to have my baby naturally at the birthing center, and now I was failing as a mother.

The midwife came in and started writing a list of what I needed to do to produce more milk. She confirmed that Baby had thrush, and while she called in a prescription to the pharmacy for both us, I nursed the baby. When I was done, the midwife re-weighed her: seven pounds, eleven ounces.

"Your baby is really okay, but still do what I wrote here because this will help you make sure you have enough milk. And so how are you? Are you eating enough?" She finally asked about me.

I broke down. She must have realized I was dealing with depression because she handed me some brochures and information about a local support group, explaining that baby blues were perfectly normal and would go away as my hormones adjusted. And that was it. When was I going to read about postpartum depression? I barely had a moment to pee, let alone try to attend a support group. Getting to our medical appointments had been stressful enough. I resisted the urge to throw the pamphlets in her face.

I cried the rest of the day at home when my husband wasn't looking. Most of the time they were silent tears. This is not what I had envisioned motherhood to be.

People wanted to come over, but that was the last thing I wanted. I couldn't stand the shame of my friends seeing my failure. The strong, independent girl they'd once known no longer lived here. She'd vanished the day my water broke. There had been no trace of her since. A broken, weepy hag with unkempt hair had replaced her. With her came this black cloud that made everything grey. Even the sun looked anemic.

Hubby told me I was doing so well. His words fell on deaf ears. "I must be doing so bad he thinks he needs to encourage me," I whispered to myself when he was out of earshot.

The next day I had my appointment with the midwife from the hospital where I had delivered. She took one look at me and asked. "How are you feeling?"

I burst into tears again. All this crying was too much for me, but I couldn't control it. I was sure someone would report me as an unfit mother and they would come take away my baby.

"Are you eating?" she asked.

I shook my head.

"Are you sleeping?"

"No," I whimpered.

She took my hand and squeezed it gently, as if to let me know she was here for me but respected my space and body. "Let's talk."

I told her how I couldn't sleep because my brain was in overload. I kept thinking about my birthing experience and what I did that made it all go wrong. How the baby was sucking the life out of me, literally. And how, just when I thought things were going better, something else would come up, like the thrush and that the other midwife thought I didn't have enough milk. And now, how I was afraid I wasn't being a good mother.

She listened patiently and calmly. In her eyes I could see she understood exactly what I was talking about and there wasn't any judgment there. When I finished my sob story, she patted my hand and said, "Let's make a plan. I want to see you next week and every week until you feel you have control once again."

The flame of hope sparked a flicker in the black fog surrounding me, and so my journey to recovery began.

CHAPTER THREE

Blessed Rest

"Get all the sleep that you can." That's what everyone and their mother kept telling me while I was pregnant, when I was in the hospital, and after I got home with my newborn. I heard it so often I thought it was some kind of inside joke that I didn't find funny.

Have any of these people had kids? I remember thinking. The answer was yes most of the time so I concluded they all were suffering from a severe case of amnesia, especially when they would ask me if I was ready for a second baby.

"You'll forget" was the response when I asked if they were kidding. Amnesia, indeed.

Lack of sleep turned out to be the biggest factor in battling postpartum depression. I asked my midwife at the two-week appointment what she meant when she said I needed to rest as much as possible.

She asked me how much sleep I usually needed in a twenty-four hour period. Eight hours usually did the trick for me.

"Then that's how much sleep you need to get, as a minimum," she said.

I laughed. "Right, and how am I supposed to accomplish this when I have to nurse every two hours around the clock?"

She smiled and patted my knee, "I didn't say all at once but added together in a twenty-four hour period, that is what you need. The baby sleeps collectively about sixteen hours a day; you need to sleep at least half that time."

If only it were that easy. I found I couldn't fall asleep so quickly. By the time I finally drifted off to la-la land, Baby would be wide awake and ready to nurse again. My brain wouldn't shut off when it was time to sleep. I would lie next to my daughter as she started sleeping for longer hours at night, watching her chest rise and fall with each little breath, obsessing about my pregnancy, labor, delivery, what went wrong, what I wished I'd done better, and so forth. As the minutes ticked by, I became so anxious and angry that I couldn't sleep. Knowing I was wasting valuable opportunities to rest only added to my frustration.

My midwife helped me with that, too. She told me to write out my birth story, pen a letter to the birthing center I had previously gone to, and keep a journal by my bed to record my thoughts, ideas, and feelings. These simple tools helped me get the tornado of thoughts out of my brain and onto paper so I didn't need to rehash the things that upset me over and over.

She also suggested sleepy-time rituals such as taking a bath, brewing a cup of relaxing tea, reading something peaceful, or doing something brainless like crocheting or filling out an easy crossword puzzle. Napping was the golden key.

"One nap a day, if not two, is a requirement," she said with a serious face. "Draw the drapes, turn off the TV, and close your eyes. If you can't fall asleep, that's okay. Just keep your eyes closed. You're still resting."

Unfortunately, with the way our house was set up, I didn't have a bed or couch to lie on except our bed. Hubby slept during the day because he worked at night, and I didn't want to disturb his sleep. We had two rocker/lounge chairs which are comfortable to rest in or watch TV, but napping or sleeping in them didn't work for me. I needed to lay flat. We moved our home around and bought a twin bed that we put in the office.

Every day when Baby took a nap in the afternoon, I would lie down next to her in the bed and snooze for a half hour. That short nap was better than a shot of espresso.

Sometimes I couldn't sleep, but I would lay there and rest or go into a deep mediation. When Baby woke up, I felt rejuvenated and ready to roll through the last leg of the day.

Over time, based on the midwife's suggestions, I developed several effective strategies to make sure I got enough quality rest:

Write it down. Keep a pad of paper, journal, or electronic tablet (that allows you to write) next to the bed. When I got ideas or thought about what I needed to do the next day, I jotted it down. Once I got it out of my brain, I didn't have to think about it again.

Relax in a Bath. "Yeah, right," I said at first. "Like I have time for that." Turns out I actually did. Maybe not for an hour-long soak, but I discovered even a fifteen or twenty minute bath could be just as beneficial, especially if I added essential oils and bath salts to the water. My favorites are lavender and chamomile oils. Organic is the best. Five to ten drops of each is plenty. For bath salts, I prefer either non-scented Epsom salts or plain Celtic sea salt. Scented salts, unless the ingredients say only essential oils were used, usually have perfumes and other harsh chemicals. Once Baby was asleep for the night, I would take fifteen minutes for a bath. Sometimes I brought a half glass of wine, a cup of sleepy tea, or a nice book. Those fifteen minutes were my "me time."

Listen to soothing music. When Baby used to be fussy at night before bedtime—the infamous witching hour—I would put the Enya station on Pandora Radio and bounce her to sleep. The quiet, relaxing music also helped lull me into a proper stupor. Whether it's classical, nature sounds, or New Age, soft music helps the brain and body relax and prepare for a long night of sleep.

Use a sound machine or white noise generator. For many people, white noise is necessary for sleep. There are many sound machines out there, ranging from $20 to $200, but a plain room fan works just fine. I found a multitude of apps for smart phones with noises from nature sounds to pink noise to jet engine. Many of them are free. Baby loved the ocean waves. I had it on her swing, and I played it on my phone at night when she had a hard time going to sleep. While the ocean put her to sleep, it also relaxed me. Eventually I bought an inexpensive sound machine so I wouldn't have to mess with my phone, which leads to the next tip.

Limit screen time. I discovered that the illuminated screen of a computer, smart phone, or TV reduces the melatonin produced naturally in the body. Melatonin is essential for a good night's sleep. I found I fell asleep easier if I avoided screen time at least an hour or two before bedtime.

Nosh on a healthy bedtime snack. Having a little bit to eat before bed helps the body relax and maintain an even blood sugar level, making it easier to stay asleep. My favorite snack is a banana and a handful of roasted nuts. Bananas contain tryptophan which helps with sleep and is a great mood booster. Nuts add an extra protein punch to help the body regenerate while resting.

Sleepy tea. There are many sleepy tea brands. My favorite brand is Traditional Medicine. I found that limiting myself to a half cup of strongly brewed tea cup prevented me from waking up to pee. Chamomile and lavender teas are good, too. Sometimes I would put a tea bag in Baby's bath at night for a light infusion of calming herbs.

Consider a dose of Calms Forte. My midwife prescribed this homeopathic medicine when I was pregnant and couldn't sleep. It didn't necessarily put me to sleep but helped relax me enough to drift into a good slumber. Calms Forte can be found at natural food stores, pharmacies, and some grocery stores.

Avoid caffeine. I know it sounds completely counterintuitive when you're sleep deprived, but I noticed that any caffeine I took, even a small cup of breakfast tea, didn't help me feel more alert. I later learned from a lecture by Dr. Sara Gottfried that coffee and other caffeinated stimulants are like a "high interest loan you have to pay back." I ended paying with less sleep at night, and the hours I did get were not quality rest.

Don't stress about not being able to sleep. I found that if I stopped obsessing about not sleeping, most of the time I fell back asleep without doing anything besides some deep breathing exercises.

Even with a well-stocked arsenal, I found it necessary to be creative. Sometimes my trusty yoga meditation CD didn't quite cut it or the cup of sleepy tea didn't sound that great on a hot summer night. My intuition played a big role in deciding what was right at certain times. Experiment to see what works best for you.

CHAPTER FOUR

Feed the Body

"Eat, you need to eat. If you don't eat, you won't produce enough milk for the baby." That's the second bit of advice people gave me constantly. The fridge was full of delicious food from friends and family. Hubby offered to cook me my favorite foods or run to the store at a moment's notice. Yet the thought of food made me nauseous, a strange feeling since I loved to eat and had readily indulged my cravings during pregnancy. Add to that the guilt and stress of knowing my not eating was affecting my baby's nutritional supply.

My midwife made a suggestion at the two-week appointment that saved my veggie bacon: "Smoothies and shakes. Drink your calories and nutrition instead of eating them if you are turned off by food right now."

And that's what I did. I bought vegetable protein powder, lots of fruit, and some leafy greens like spinach and kale. The Christmas before Baby was born, we had gifted ourselves a new Vitamix blender—simply the best present we could have purchased. Vitamix blenders are easy to use and clean, which is what you need when you're short on time. Within two to three minutes, I had a nutrient-packed, yummy-tasting smoothie and a clean blender. No fussing around. A good quality blender is the key. Plus, you can use it later for making healthy baby food.

I played around with the ingredients but made sure I had protein, greens, and vitamin C in every smoothie. Protein provides strength and energy. Greens provide necessary fiber and folic acid to help with digestion and prevent constipation. Dark-green leafy foods also have calcium to replenish the body's supply while you are breastfeeding. Vitamin C boosts the immune system and helps with recovery.

During the first month postpartum, one of my "mama" friends brought me a bag of goodies. Inside were energy bars, fruit, bottled smoothies, and cheese. She said this was a sample of what she kept on hand for when she didn't have time to sit down and eat a meal. That bag of goodies was the best food gift anyone could have given me. All the yummy cooked food in the fridge required that it be put in a serving dish and heated in the microwave. I didn't have time for that or the dirty dishes afterward. An energy bar with a piece of fruit or a cheese stick came in handy when I needed to eat something but didn't have time for a sit-down meal. The sampling of healthy snacking food gave me an idea for what to shop for at the grocery store.

The protein bars were *Lara Bar* brand, which are gluten free and made of whole ingredients without preservatives. In addition to tasting delicious, these bars are a great source of protein and come in a variety of flavors.

The bottles of smoothies were *Naked* brand. *Odwalla* has some great smoothies, too. They have an awesome green one with spirulina and are packed with lots of super fruits and veggies. These bottled smoothies are a great alternative for busy moms who don't have a blender, limited time, and while on the go.

A Russian friend, who also happened to be a doula, brought me a couple bottles of kefir shortly after I came home from the hospital and was dealing with thrush. She told me that in Russia they give mothers kefir to drink after birth every day. I didn't realize why it was so good until I had the thrush problem. Kefir contains anywhere from twelve up to fifty different probiotic organisms—three times or more than plain yogurt—that are essential for fighting infections, especially yeast. These microbes provide vital support to the immune system and help with digestion. A cup a day is my usual "dose." I love to add it to my smoothies.

When I returned to work, I discovered I had even less time in the kitchen. But I still needed to eat. Snack food didn't quite cut it anymore. After brainstorming, I discovered I needed to cook. Cook! I know that's a scary word for some, but hear me out.

There are many easy, quick, nutritious recipes that provide the sustenance needed for a breastfeeding mom. I invested in a quality set of glass storage containers able to hold two to three servings each. Glass is best because are no worries about plastic leaching into food during microwaving. After I prepared an entree, I filled these containers, along with a side dish. For example, lasagna made with vegetarian protein got a side of steamed broccoli or carrots. Voilà! Carbs, veggies, and protein all in one container, ready to heat and eat.

To avoid eating the same dish several days in a row, I stored extra portions in the freezer. When I needed a quick meal, all I had to do was pull a container out, let it defrost, and then heat.

I used this same "make-ahead" strategy for salads, also. Toss desired ingredients into separate containers (minus dressing) and then assemble when needed. When you are done eating, all you have to do is put the container in the dishwasher.

Creating healthy grab-and-go meals not only helped me maintain good nutrition while my body healed from the childbirth, but it also saved money and time. I kept a container of peeled and cut carrots for snacking, a bowl of hard-boiled eggs for an extra protein punch during the day, and hummus in the fridge. Sometimes I only had a couple of minutes to grab a bite so I tried to make that snack as hardy as possible because it might be a while before I could eat again.

During the first couple of months when I was nursing around the clock, I kept a sealed container with crackers, walnuts, and dried fruit next to my bed for midnight snacks. Low blood sugar affects sleep and having something there that can satisfy middle-of-the-night hunger without having to get up out of bed was great for helping me get back to sleep.

Here are a few of the quick and easy recipes I use often:

Garbanzo Spinach Salad

1 can of garbanzo beans or 2 cups of cooked garbanzo beans
3 cups of spinach, cut (I like to use baby spinach)
1-2 yellow pepper (chopped)
1-2 roasted red peppers (chopped)
1 small onion (chopped)
2-3 tbsp. extra virgin olive oil
1 tbsp. balsamic vinegar

1 fresh squeezed lemon
Salt and pepper to taste
Mix all of the vegetables in a large bowl. Sprinkle salt and pepper to taste. Drizzle oil, vinegar, and lemon juice. Mix well. Refrigerate for twelve hours. Serve cold.

Southwest Quinoa Salad

1 cup quinoa (cooked)
1 bundle cilantro (chopped)
1 small onion (chopped)
1 cup cooked yellow corn
1 cup cooked black beans
1 large red pepper (chopped)
1 yellow pepper (chopped)
1 fresh squeezed lime
2-3 tbsp. extra virgin olive oil
Salt and pepper to taste
1 sliced avocado
1 jalapeno pepper (chopped) *optional
Mix all of the vegetables. Sprinkle salt and pepper to taste. Drizzle with oil and lime juice. Mix well. Refrigerate for twelve hours. Serve cold with sliced avocado.

Power Green Smoothie

1 cup spinach
1 apple
1 fresh squeezed lemon or 2 fresh squeezed oranges
1 cucumber
¼- ½ avocado

1 scoop protein powder of choice
Blend until smooth. You can also add milk for extra calcium. I prefer almond or soy milk and sometimes I add my daily cup of kefir.

Very Berry Smoothie

1 banana
½ cup blueberries
½ cup strawberries
½ cup raspberries
¼ cup black currents
1 scoop protein powder of choice
Milk to desired smoothness
Blend until smooth. I like to use either fresh or frozen berries. Berries are high in antioxidants, which boost the immune system and help recovery from delivery.

You've heard the phrase "you are what you eat." Well, it's true. Eat healthy, strong foods and your body will be healthy and strong. Not only that, but you'll be providing yummy nutrition to your little one. Remember organic is best.

Rachael Ray has lots of great, quick recipes on her website that take thirty minutes or less. I go there a lot for inspiration.

CHAPTER FIVE

Pampering Time

The hospital midwife continued to give suggestions on things I could do to improve my sleep and feel better. Go outside. Take a bath. Light a candle and have a moment alone. "Self-care, self-care, self-care," she repeated.

"Yeah, right!" I laughed.

"I'm serious. You need to take good care of yourself if you want to be there for your girl," she said in a firm but gentle voice.

As I listened to her, I saw a glimmer of hope for the first time in two weeks even if I didn't quite feel it. She watched me nurse Baby and said I was doing fine and not to worry. When I got home that afternoon, I called the birthing center and canceled the rest of my postpartum appointments with them—a painful thing to do because I adored my original midwife. But I needed to get my care from a place where I felt better supported. I also had too many dark memories of my labor at the birthing center and with everything going on, I didn't have time to heal those wounds yet.

The next day I had Baby's two-week appointment with the pediatrician. They said her weight was fine and that I had a perfect baby—music to my heart. Maybe I wasn't the worst mother in the world. I didn't realize how much I depended on external validation until that moment.

That week I started to apply the tools the midwife had given me. Hubby watched Baby after I nursed her one morning so I could take a bath. I went all out—lighting candles, dumping in Celtic sea salts, and sprinkling the water with essential oils of lavender and tangerine. I never wanted to leave the tub once I got in.

As I lay in the tub, I realized there is always time for self-care. It didn't have to be an hour-long Swedish massage or a deep pore-cleansing facial, although those are quite nice and every mother deserves special treatment.

I learned never to underestimate the benefit of basic hygiene. The first time my daughter sat in the bouncy seat on the bathroom floor while I took a shower was a huge breakthrough for me. Up to that point, I waited for my husband to get home from work or be home to watch her so I could shower. Now I felt empowered, like, "I can do this mother thing. You just watch me."

Self-care was as simple as taking five minutes to pluck my eyebrows or paint my toenails. I was amazed how great I felt for doing something nice for myself. Every time I looked down at my feet and saw the pretty pink polish twinkling in the light, I had a smile on my face. A smiling mama leads to a happy mama, which then in turn leads to a happy home.

I know there are mamas out there that feel guilty for even thinking they want a little self-care or wish they could take a break and get a pedicure at a salon. Release the guilt, ladies. There is absolutely no reason for it. We deserve the time for ourselves.

We deserve to have some "me time" and even spend some money on ourselves. After all, we are the queens of the household, and it's okay to look the part.

I finally got over myself and realized it was okay to hand the baby to my husband when he walked through the door and to let him know I needed a half hour to take a bath or read a favorite book or go in the other room and close the door for some quiet time. I know some moms feel bad handing their little one to their partners because said partner has been working all day and is tired. Well, guess what? Parenting is a team effort. It took two to bring that precious life into this world. They're not going to die if they need to hold a baby for a half hour so Mom can recharge. If your spouse is unavailable, call a friend or a family member to come over for a while.

Take time today to do something nice for yourself, dear mothers. What are five quick things you can do for yourself that would make you happy? Write them down and tape that list to your bathroom mirror to remind yourself that you are worth making time for.

Here are some ideas of things I came up with to nurture myself:

Take a bath.

Have a glass of wine or a cup of tea.

Take time to shave or wax.

Take an extra-long shower and use my favorite conditioner.

Make a decadent cup of hot chocolate complete with chocolate sprinkles or marshmallows.

Brush and style my hair as if going to a fancy dinner or on a date with Brad Pitt.

Apply my favorite makeup.

Get a massage or facial.

Soak my feet in Epsom salt bath and favorite essential oils.

Visit with a friend over lunch or coffee. (This is extra special if you can leave the baby with your partner or a trusted babysitter.)

Go for a walk. I used to walk down to the local park and bring a book. Baby would fall asleep on the way so when we got to the park, I would find a nice shady bench and read for a half hour while she slept—my favorite kind of me time.

Go shopping and buy some flowers.

Put on my favorite music and dance. Dancing is a great way to exercise and quite a mood booster. Any time I'm feeling down and I can't seem to shake it off, I literally have to shake it to get back on track.

Read a book or magazine.

There are so many things to do in a few minutes that can lift your spirit and revitalize your soul. A great book I found on self-care is *The Art of Extreme Self-care* by Cheryl Richardson. It's not being selfish taking time to do something nice for you. The better you care for yourself, the better mother you'll be. My midwife was totally right.

CHAPTER SIX

Processing and Reflection

Probably the best piece of advice I received from my midwife was to sit down and write my birth story. For most mothers, the first birth never goes the way they anticipated. One of the common themes I heard from birth stories is that the first child came with lots of drama. Mothers who intended to have natural births ended up with interventions, C-sections, complications they wanted to avoid. These moms usually share that it was the birth of their second child that brought healing or gave them the desired birth story they dreamed of.

Well, that's sweet and all, but in my situation, I wasn't planning on having a second child, but I needed healing, too. I first wrote out my birth story and posted it to my blog. I left out some of the emotional things I went through because I didn't think anyone wanted to hear that. Then I wrote an email to my first midwife from the birthing center, explaining my disappointment with the outcome of my experience and the way things had been handled at the birthing center. She forwarded my email to the director, who then called me. We talked and I was able to tell her my side of the story and give suggestions of how things could have been dealt with in my situation as feedback for future clients. She was kind and very understanding. Because she listened to me as I voiced my concerns, I was able to heal those wounds and move forward. Months later I was able to stop by the center and bring lunch to the midwife and assistants—something that gave me positive closure.

I also called a friend who had a one and a half year old. We talked for an hour. More accurately I talked. She listened but did mention to me how she had felt those first couple of weeks. She said to hang in there because it does get better.

By the third week postpartum, my perineum hurt less. At least it didn't feel like I was spraying turpentine on an open wound every time I peed and it didn't itch anymore. The pain had started to subside slightly. I took a nap every day, and I started to feel a little more human. One day I actually put my contacts in and normal clothes on. I actually started to let people come over to visit.

Mama friends came by and confirmed that the first month for them had been hell also, but if I could just hold on, things would get easier. I took their words to heart, especially when Hubby went back to work.

I stressed out about him being gone at night, even though Baby had been sleeping pretty well. I was certain that once he left for work, she would start crying and I wouldn't be able to handle her. We'd watched the *Purple Crying Period* DVD the hospital gave us when we went home, and I silently freaked out about not being able to take care of my baby alone. Up to this point when she had crying periods, he'd been there to help me or take turns bouncing her.

The first night alone, she fussed but went to sleep within a half hour and slept for three or four hours between feedings. I didn't sleep as well because I worried, but we survived the night. Eventually I got used to Hubby not being there and was able to sleep more.

Although I started feeling better, my appetite still hadn't returned. I remember coming from an appointment and we drove by Burgerville, a Pacific Northwest fast food chain. "I think I'm craving a milk shake," I said. Hubby steered across lanes of traffic into the drive-thru without a second thought. If I hinted that I might want something, he made sure I had it.

Within a month, I started to get more cravings for food and actually ate an entire meal for the first time since I'd delivered our daughter. She also started to sleep on her own without me holding her and spending awake time in places other than my arms. Sometimes she would sit in her swing up to twenty minutes. I remember the first time she did that. I ran around the house like a tornado. Pee, eat, load the dishwasher, finish the laundry, brush teeth, wash face, brush hair, change clothes, sweep the floor, and respond to some text messages—I did all that in twenty minutes.

At six months postpartum, I reached a very low point where nothing seemed to work. I had gone back to work but was able to work from home most of the week. This came as both a curse and blessing. I know thousands of mothers who would kill to have a job that allows them to stay home and care for their little ones, but it's a lot harder than it sounds. The older my daughter got, the more demanding she became. A large portion of my job required full concentration—something I couldn't give with a sleep-deprived brain and a crying infant on my lap.

I dared not complain because I wanted to work from home and had advocated this benefit with great zeal during my pregnancy. Wouldn't want to sound ungrateful now, would I? I trudged on, day after day, like a zombie, going through the motions, but never really registering what I was doing.

It was in the midst of this slog of despair that I started writing this book. I needed to write down what helped me in months prior, not only so I could come back and reference those tips again, but also to share my experience of what I was going through. At the time I felt so isolated. Sure, most of my friends where working moms, but most of them had either parents helping them out by babysitting or their kids were in daycare. None of them worked full-time and cared for their infant simultaneously.

A typical day for me was getting up at three-thirty in the morning after nursing my daughter, clocking in, making a cup of breakfast tea, and logging into the remote desktop at work. After two hours of working hard, Baby would wake up and want to nurse again. Most of the time she went back to sleep, but sometimes she didn't so I would then place her in the baby carrier on my chest and bounce on the yoga ball at my desk as I continued to work.

Sometime around seven-thirty or eight, Hubby would come home from work, and he would take her for a couple of hours while I worked on the tasks that required the most focus. When it was time for him to go to bed, I would take her again and continue bouncing on the yoga ball or she would sit in the swing for up to forty-five minutes. Sometimes she would lie in the bassinet next to my desk. With one hand on her belly and one hand on the keyboard, I would continue to work until she got tired of lying there. And then there was all the nursing, diaper changing, and burping in between. Honestly I have no idea how I met my required weekly and monthly goals with all of the interruptions. Looking back, I'm amazed I was able to keep my job. At two-thirty in the afternoon, I would clock out. The first thing I would do is try to nap with Baby. The rest of the day was pure survival mode. The simplest tasks felt like massive mountains to be climbed so I just stuck to what was absolutely necessary. Laundry and dishes were only done when I ran out of utensils or underwear, housecleaning went out the window, and connecting with friends in person or via social media became ancient history. I spent the rest of the day rocking Baby, staring at the images on TV until Hubby got up to go to work. That was my cue that it was bedtime.

Bathe, nurse, lay Baby in bed, fifteen-minute bath for me, and then pass out until she woke up a couple of hours later and then another couple of hours after that. Repeat until three-thirty in the morning and start all over again.

For the first time, I understood why some moms looked forward to going to work. When my one day in the office arrived each week, I cherished that day like a priceless family heirloom gem. But the office day didn't always feel like an escape. For the first three months after returning to work, I had to pump every three hours during my ten-hour shift, which meant all my breaks were dedicated to milk production. I could never fully get away from being a mother. It was hard not to feel bitter. Or guilty for feeling bitter.

I turned to my journal, writing these things down. I knew I would need a therapist soon, and my memory was so gone that I wouldn't remember specifics if I didn't write them down. I also got over not telling people how I felt. When they asked me how it was going I said, "Terrible. This whole mother-work thing sucks ass."

I yelled a lot. Mostly at myself, but occasionally at my daughter when she wouldn't stop crying or go to sleep. This rage inside would make me feel like the stinkiest piece of shit mom on the planet. How could a mother scream and curse at her own offspring? That only made her cry more, for obvious reasons, and then I felt worse. Sometimes I wanted to slap her. The first time that thought crossed my mind, I immediately placed her in the bassinet and went into the other room. *Oh god, I knew now how child abuse happens.* It took every ounce of will power to walk away, even if I left her screaming her head off. There were so many times the thought of throwing her against the wall would hit me like a tidal wave. Every time I had to put her down and walk away because I was afraid I'd actually do it.

Sometimes I would down a half glass of wine and step outside on the balcony for a few seconds to take a breather; other times I put my headphones on and cranked up some death metal song until my ears would ring. I always felt more in control afterward, and she calmed down when I picked her up the second time. Each time this happened, guilt and relief would dance a wicked tango inside my gut. I walked a fine line, and I knew it.

Writing, talking, and sharing were all part of the processing I needed. By writing these things down, it allowed my brain to take a break from rehashing the scenario over and over in my head while I was lying awake in bed, not sleeping. Once I documented my birth story and wrote the email to the birthing center midwife, I started to sleep better.

I encourage every new mom to get a journal and jot down their story or type it out on the computer. Write all the things you loved, the things you hated, the things you wished you had done, and all your emotions surrounding your birth. Don't hold back. Even if it's messy and sounds depressing, get it out. The sooner you process it, the sooner you can begin to heal.

CHAPTER SEVEN

Bump in the Road

Hubby did our taxes several weeks after the birth of our daughter and it turned out we would be receiving a refund that would cover most of the hospital bill. Between the partial refund from the birthing center, tax return, and a generous financial gift from a family member, we managed to pay the insurance deductibles and have enough money for bills while on unpaid maternity leave. That relieved much of the stress.

Little by little, the grey fog slowly dissipated and I could see sunshine again. I also discovered my parents were a huge help. Once or twice a week, I would drive three hours roundtrip to see them when Hubby was working. Baby slept the whole way, which was a nice change. When I arrived at their country cottage, I would nurse my daughter and then hand her over to Grandma and Grandpa. I'd slip into their room and take a two-hour nap. A healthy, tasty vegan meal awaited me when I woke up. Grandparents got baby time, Mommy got sleep, and Grandma got to feed her daughter nutritious food which made Grandma feel useful—a win-win for all.

A month and a half postpartum, I felt great. I went in for my six-week appointment with the hospital midwife and was excited about getting an IUD. However, the moment she started inserting the speculum, I about leapt off the table. My bottom hadn't healed completely, and the metal rubbing against the small raw wound felt like I was going to tear again. The midwife said to come back in two weeks to have my condition reevaluated.

I was crushed. When I went home, I pulled an old mirror out for the first time since I delivered and checked out what had happened down there. Tears spilled down my cheeks as I sat on the edge of the bathtub in horror.

Nothing looked right. Flaps of skin that looked like hemorrhoids filled the space between my vagina and anus. Right above the vagina, a weird-looking structure appeared, which later I learned was a cystocele. I didn't remember seeing that there before. My clitoris looked like a tiny nub swallowed up by the still-swollen outer labial folds. Every time I touched it when I adjusted my underwear or washed down there, it throbbed and not in a good way. No wonder sex was the last thing on my mind. Not only was I not interested, now I felt violated and deformed. Damaged. Would I ever be able to have sex again? Or even enjoy it?

Hubby kept telling me I was beautiful and very sexy, especially since my breasts had grown from a small A cup to a voluptuous B-borderline-C. He said that all of the changes in my female organs didn't matter to him. He loved the new me just as much as before, actually even more after what I went through to birth our gorgeous little girl. These words fell on deaf ears. No matter what he said, I didn't feel sexy. Yes, I did feel his love and I knew he wouldn't leave me, but I couldn't help but feel inadequate.

That day I went onto Facebook to escape my dismal reality. On the right-hand side of the screen where the advertisements are located, I saw an ad for *Oprah &The Chopra Center 21-day Meditation Challenge* for *Perfect Health*. It intrigued me, but I didn't click on it. A week later when I logged back in on one of the pages I follow, *Fit Mom*, she posted a journal entry from her experience with the meditation challenge. In her post, she mentioned how lovely it was for her to have twenty minutes of alone time because her child had been sick and attached to her all day.

This struck a chord with me. My child wasn't ill, but at this stage in her life, she was practically attached to my chest, either sleeping or nursing.

I found the page for the challenge and signed up, even though it had started over a week earlier. I did two meditations a day to get caught up. Sometimes I was alone and sometimes I did them at night while my daughter slept next to me. Each one brought a sense of peace and tranquility to my chaotic introduction to motherhood.

A week later, I went back to the hospital midwife. With the aid of a lot of numbing gel and deep breathing (thanks to the meditation I'd been doing) on my part, we got the IUD in. Oh. My. God! It hurt, but after what I went through eight weeks prior, I knew I never wanted to experience that kind of pain ever again so I put up with the crampy, stabby pain the IUD gave me. According to the midwife, this was normal and would subside after a couple of days.

Well, it didn't. Six days later, I woke up with incredible pain. It felt like needles were moving around inside my pelvis.

I would be lying motionless in bed and the breathtaking jolty pain would come out of nowhere and then disappear. Sometime it would come when I moved, but there wasn't any specific pattern. Up to this point, I'd been bleeding and I hadn't bothered to check the strings of the IUD. I did that morning. I didn't feel anything, but then I wasn't sure what I was looking for in the first place.

I called the midwife, and she had me come in. The pelvic exam she did about killed me. It was all I could do to not to scream or kick her in the face. Memories of my labor came flooding back. She couldn't find the strings, and this concerned her greatly. She sent me to the emergency room across the street for an ultrasound. The whole time I had my daughter with me because we were supposed to meet up with out-of-town relatives for a visit. I called my husband who had worked the entire night before and asked him to come to the ER.

When he arrived, they were about to do the ultrasound, using a transvaginal probe. They had barely inserted the probe and I screamed. My whole body shook as my vision blurred and I closed my legs as tight as possible. I remember thinking, "This must be what rape victims go through every time they get a pelvic exam." I knew they needed to do the ultrasound so I let them drug me. Even through my pharmaceutically induced haze, I still felt the pain as the technician stretched my vaginal opening to manipulate the probe. Silent tears fell from my eyes. *Please don't rip again.*

To make matters worse, they couldn't find the IUD. I went through all of that for nothing, at least that's how it felt. They brought in a portable x-ray machine and took a picture of my pelvic and lower abdominal area. Sure enough, they found the IUD. It was hanging out on the right side, next to my uterus.

"Well, you know what this means," the ER doctor said, with a sympathetic look on his face. "You're going to need surgery."

I sighed. "Yes."

Since I'd eaten at twelve-thirty, they said they couldn't do the surgery until eight-thirty that evening. It was four-thirty.

I turned to my very tired husband. "You need to take the baby home before you are too exhausted to drive. I'll be okay." I put on a stoic face, even though every fiber in my body wanted him to stay with me. But having a two-month-old in the hospital wouldn't be fun for any of the parties involved. "I'll call Missy or Sarah."

"Okay," he replied reluctantly. He clearly didn't want to leave either, but it wasn't about us anymore. We had a baby to think about.

While we waited for the surgeon to come talk to me, I called my two friends. They both dropped everything and came over right away. One girlfriend's husband was out of town and she had to get a sitter for her son while the other was in the middle of moving.

I nursed Baby before my husband left. Suddenly the room that had been bustling with nurses, doctors, and technicians felt deserted. With no one there to distract me, I expected my emotions to erupt like an angry volcano, but instead, I lay there quietly in shock, contemplating what had just happened.

I'd been excited that I had birth control and had been cleared to exercise. I could finally return to some sort of normalcy and then this. Why? Why Universe? Is this karmic punishment for not being strong enough to deliver my daughter naturally? For not recycling enough? Or not using cloth diapers right away like I had planned?

Before I could really get myself further down the rabbit hole of suck, the surgeon came in to talk to me. He turned out to be the same physician who had done the vacuum extraction for my baby. Relief washed over me like a soothing warm shower. At least I would be in good hands.

"We need to stop meeting like this." He smiled. "How is your little girl?"

"Growing like a weed." I managed a smile.

We chatted a bit before he broke the news. "I'm not actually going to be doing the surgery. My shift is over in a half hour, but Dr. X will take over. She'll take really good care of you."

Damn. A tidal wave of disappointment ended my short-lived respite of relief. Sarah showed up while the doctor talked to me. She could sense my deflated spirit and took my hand in hers. When the physician left, I nearly broke down but Sarah's sweet energy kept me strong.

The nurse came in shortly and started an IV bag of fluids I'd need before surgery and put in a catheter. Dear Lord, that didn't feel good. The only thing left to do before they took me to the operating room was to put the compression stockings on my legs.

Missy arrived shortly after the nurse left. Having my goddess sisters there gave me courage and buoyed my spirits. I was about to experience the first surgery of my life, but I didn't feel too nervous because those two wonderful women were there.

Dr. X came in to see me right before eight. She was a youthful blond who looked too young to be operating on me.

"So when are you doing this surgery?" I asked.

She pursed her lips. "Uh, not tonight, if that's what you were expecting."

"What?" I whispered.

"You are an urgent case, not an emergency," she said. "Emergencies come first and then we'll fit you in."

"Excuse me?" Missy folded her arms across her chest and leaned against the bed on my left. "She's been waiting for this surgery for hours while in pain."

"How can a perforated IUD floating around in her abdomen not be an emergency?" Sarah placed her hand on my right shoulder.

Did I mention how much I loved these two ladies?

"It hasn't perforated her bowel or bladder so she's okay. If it had, we'd have wheeled her in to the OR when she first arrived," the doctor explained.

"Oh, so we're going to wait until it does?" one of my friends asked.

"Of course not. We can keep her here overnight to manage her pain, and we'll see when we can get her in tomorrow. Or she can go home and call my office to have them schedule the surgery so we'll have a certain time."

One of the girls said something, but I didn't hear anything else as everything inside me collapsed. The sliver of hope I'd felt the last couple of days vanished as the dark fog settled in once again. I couldn't believe this was happening to me. I was relieved Sarah and Missy were there to speak for me because I had no words. They knew me well and weren't afraid to speak up for me. Missy told the doctor I needed a moment to powwow with my girls.

After the surgeon left, Missy suggested that I go home since it looked like they were going to send me home anyway and call my OB in the morning to schedule me at my preferred hospital. She thought I would be more comfortable having my doctor operate on me than this woman. She was right.

Ten hours after I'd walked into the ER, I went home, still in pain but with a prescription for strong pain meds.

First thing the following morning, I called the OB office. Dr. D was out of town but his partner, Dr. B, was available to do the surgery. She was the doctor I wanted originally when I found out I was pregnant and this pleased me greatly. She had me come in that afternoon for a pre-op visit.

When she went to do the pelvic exam, I cringed, waiting for the pain to hit when she inserted the speculum. It never came. I felt her prodding around, but her touch was so gentle and she used a very small speculum to avoid causing me anymore discomfort.

"Your perineum hasn't healed, honey. That's why you're in so much pain. Have you been referred for pelvic physical therapy?" Dr. B asked, while examining me.

"I've never heard of that, so no."

"I read your hospital record. You had a long labor. For all of my patients that had long labor or tore, I refer them to pelvic PT." She went on to explain, "This is a unique therapy for the pelvic area to deal with discomfort and help you get back to a normal life, including intimacy."

"Really?" Tiny seeds of hope sprouted in my heart, despite the dark fog.

"Yes." She covered me back up when she finished the exam. She pointed at my abdomen and showed me where the incisions would be. "If there isn't any damage to your other organs, the surgery will only take about thirty to forty minutes. I'm also going to give you a small tube of estrogen cream. Apply that to you perineal area to help speed up the healing."

For the first time since I delivered my baby, I felt that maybe, just maybe, I could actually get some of my life back. I suddenly wished I had stayed with this OB clinic to begin with and wondered how my birth story would have turned out if I'd listened to my gut. But you can't change the past and since I planned on only having one child, there wouldn't be another next time unless the universe had a different plan for me. I knew one thing as I mourned my poor decision; I would continue my women's health care with this doctor from now on.

The surgery was scheduled for the following morning. I checked in at six and Missy drove me home before noon. It pretty much was a non-event. I hurt for about four days but healed pretty quickly. I spent most of my recovery period at my parents' place so they could help me with the baby because Hubby had to work. He didn't have any vacation left to take since he'd used it up with Baby at the beginning of my maternity leave.

At my two-week post-op appointment, Dr. B cleared me to return to normal activity. I could start swimming and working out. She also gave me a referral to have pelvic PT. That was the beginning of my second recovery.

CHAPTER EIGHT

Moving the Body

Before I got pregnant, I hated working out or going to the gym. I stayed active by hiking, skiing, and kayaking, but didn't make much effort in keeping up with my level of fitness. The week after I found out I was pregnant, I joined the gym. I wanted a natural birth and getting my butt in shape was mandatory.

Through the first trimester, I swam for thirty minutes every day, four to five times a week in the morning before work. This helped me with morning sickness a lot. Then I got lazy after I started feeling better. But as I entered my third trimester, I went back to the pool, mainly because it felt wonderful letting the water support my growing belly. I loved being in the water, and swimming didn't feel like a workout. I also did a couple of online prenatal yoga videos.

After the baby came, my exercise routine came to a halt. First of all, I hurt. Every time I stood longer than a few minutes, I felt like all my internal organs were going to collapse through my vagina. The only exercise I got was bouncing Baby on the yoga ball when she fussed. The IUD incident set me back another three weeks before I was cleared to go back to the gym. Finally, after almost three months, I hit the pool. It felt so wonderful, cutting through the water from one end of the pool to the other. I also started to do the yoga classes they offered at my gym. I did a little yoga with the baby at home when I couldn't make it to the gym.

Fifteen minutes a day I did a few exercises on the floor with Baby. Slowly my body started to trim up and return to the shape it was before I got pregnant. I felt great. That's what exercise does. It releases endorphins through the body making you feel good—an excellent way to fight depression.

All went well until I started working full-time again. Since we didn't have childcare (because I worked from home mostly), all of the time Hubby was available to watch Baby was dedicated to my working hours. I had also started pelvic physical therapy and was getting acupuncture to help with pain in my body. Gym time went by the wayside and so did my fifteen minutes of yoga with Baby.

After a month of not working out, I realized I needed to do something because depression set in once again. Working at a computer forty hours a week didn't help.

I discovered that for ten extra dollars a month, I could bring my baby to the gym and put her in the kids' club. At first, I didn't want to do that because I couldn't stand the thought of some stranger watching my baby while I did the downward facing dog in the other room, but I talked to the girls who worked in the kids' club and checked out the area where they kept the babies.

I learned that the people who work in these childcare facilities are trained professionals. They know what to do in case of an emergency; they like kids and are great with them.

I was only going to leave her there for an hour or two at most and if there was a problem, they would come find me in the gym. I was in the same building, after all. It took me months to finally let go of my fears and embrace the fact that I had this wonderful opportunity to exercise and enjoy some baby-free time. I decided to bite the bullet and do it.

The first time I took her was a Sunday morning. Of course, when I got there I thought she might have filled her drawers. It turned out to be a false alarm. She then upchucked a fair amount of her feeding all over my tank top. At this point, I'd been procrastinating so much about bringing her to the gym that this only made me want to take her home and skip the class, but I resisted the urge to rush out to the car and strap her back into the car seat.

I ended up being late for class but was so happy I went. Every pose and stretch brought joy to my body, even though I'd get whiffs of regurgitated milk every so often. Bringing my baby to the gym allowed me the freedom to exercise when I wanted and gave me some much needed "me" time.

With that being said, I found I didn't have to join the gym to exercise or have someone watch Baby so I could work out. She really enjoyed the time I stretched and did yoga poses on the floor with her. She giggled every time I did push-ups over her because when I came down, I would kiss her belly before pumping back up. My local library carried a variety of "baby and me" yoga books which I took full advantage of during the first six months.

We also took walks. Lots of them! Sometimes I would put her in the baby carrier on my chest or in the stroller. Walking was a gentle way to move my body and a great weight-bearing exercise. But I found the following five exercises were the easiest to incorporate into my daily routine:

Pushups. They strengthen your arms, back, abs, and core. And they can be done anywhere.

Reverse pushups. They work the triceps. It's very important that this set of muscles gets worked because they support the biceps, which are used when you carry your baby.

Walking. Unless you are in a wheelchair, anyone can walk. Walking gave me time to think, fresh air, and a chance to exercise. I always felt better after a walk, even if it was just around the block.

Crunches. I love these because they can be done anywhere. In yoga class, the instructor had me lift my legs and bend the knees while lying on my back as if sitting in a chair. With laced hands behind head, I inhaled and then exhaled as I brought my chin to chest. Sometimes I added a pumping action of my legs like riding a bicycle and a twist bringing the elbow to the opposite knee (right elbow to left knee and left elbow to right knee).

Bridges. This is a fun exercise I learned from a mom and baby yoga video. I'd lay on my back with bent knees, keeping feet flat on the ground and Baby on tummy facing me (tummy-to-tummy). On the inhale, I'd lift my butt off the ground high enough until my body was a nice long plane from knees to chest. The baby slid down until her face touched mine. I'd hold for four seconds and then lower back down. This resulted in lots of baby giggles, which was so much better than crying.

No matter what I did, I noticed that the more I moved my body the better I felt the rest of the day. Sometimes it meant just turning up my favorite dance song and getting my groove on in the living room. When the gym wasn't an option, I found workout videos online or from the local library. YouTube has an abundance of exercise videos ranging from five minutes to an hour.

CHAPTER NINE

Going Within

I've been meditating for several years now. Okay, maybe I should rephrase that. I've been learning how to meditate for a long time. Sometimes I get it right and I fall into a wonderful trance for a good thirty minutes. Those days, however, tend to be far and few in between. It wasn't until I did the *Oprah & Chopra Center 21-Day Perfect Health Meditation* challenge that I finally realized a five to ten minute meditation can be just as effective as an hour-long session. Sure, if you have the time and can do it for thirty minutes or more, great! But nobody knows better than a mom how difficult it is to even find time to go use the bathroom, let alone take a half hour to zone out.

I'm here to tell you that both are possible. It all depends on how you prioritize your "spare" time. Some moms prefer to fold laundry or clean the bathroom when the baby is napping because if the laundry isn't put away or the toilet isn't clean, they'll lose the delicate hold on their fragile sanity. I tend to fall into that category to a certain extent, but I discovered awareness is sort of like a meditation which means while I'm pulling out that toilet brush or folding my daughter's adorable little onesies, I can still meditate.

That's right. I learned to practice deep breathing as I placed each article of clothing into the laundry basket. I felt the softness and smelled the freshness of the fabric. I blessed each outfit and imagined threads of white protective light weaving through the seams, a purple shielding light to protect my little one from harsh energy, a green healing light to help her with the upset tummy issue she'd been having, and a calm loving pink light to sooth her throughout the day.

While scrubbing away the mineral buildup in the toilet bowel, I visualized those areas inside myself that could use a little scouring. Most of the time it was guilt for not doing something "the right way" or getting down on myself for not always being the world's best mom. Those icky energies needed to be cleaned out. So when I finished scrubbing and flushed the filth down the drain, I visualized an energetic flushing of the things I no longer wished to carry.

Those were just a few ways to make the simplest task a beautiful spiritual experience that left me refreshed and brought awareness into my daily life. Awareness cultivates a deeper sense of calm. At first it seemed like work, but I just stuck to one task a day and the more I practiced this, the easier it became.

I also learned in this process that I could actually take time to meditate sitting cross-legged on a pillow with a candle burning in front of me and Tibetan bowls music playing in the background while I closed my eyes and said "Om" over and over. Well, I didn't actually do all that, but you get my point.

Here's how it worked for me. My baby napped for a half hour so I would take five to ten minutes of that half hour to meditate. I'd find a quiet place, somewhere near Baby so I could hear her if she woke up. Sometimes I would put on relaxing ambient music or nature sounds. The music also helped her sleep better, which meant a longer nap time.

Here's a quick meditation that could be done in five to twenty minutes—it all depends on how long you want to stay in it.

Find a place to relax. Whether it's sitting or lying down or lounging on the couch or recliner. Wherever it is, make sure you are comfortable and the temperature is right. Before you begin your meditation, it's very helpful to make sure your basic bodily needs are met so get a drink of water or use the bathroom. Close your eyes and let's begin.

Take a couple deep breaths by inhaling slowly and counting to five as you exhale. After your second or third breath, imagine as you inhale that you are breathing in fresh air as if you are outside somewhere in nature. You are in your favorite natural retreat near a body of water. You can hear that water lapping at your feet. Whether it is a roaring ocean or babbling brook, when the water touches your feet it feels cool and refreshing.

With each wave, imagine the glistening, pure water flowing up over your body, washing your entire being. As it cascades down from the top of your head, visualize it cleansing your crown chakra, leaving it as a brilliant white diamond, the third eye chakra an amethyst, the throat chakra a sapphire, the heart chakra an emerald or rose quartz, the solar plexus chakra a citrine, the naval chakra a carnelian, and your root chakra a ruby. The water carries away any impurities or negative energies that may have latched on to your energy centers. The body of water absorbs these and you are now clean and refreshed.

Wiggle your toes and feel the earth below you. You feel the ground sink slightly as your feet anchor into the earth grounding you. Feel the deep energy of the planet holding you, supporting you as you stand there. You are mother and you are connected to the Mother. She nourishes and protects you. She guides and gives you the strength you need for today and all your tomorrows.

Look up to the sky and feel the warmth of the sun radiating down upon you. Imagine that the cells of your skin are like millions of tiny solar panels absorbing the energy from the sun. All the energy flows into your solar plexus, your internal sun, charging your batteries up. As they charge, know you can never have too much or too little energy. Your core and power center will always have access to this sun to charge whenever needed.

A gentle wind blows across your face and envelopes your entire body in warmth. The air surrounding you carries the promise of hope and reminds you to be gentle with yourself, dear one. You have the wisdom and resourcefulness to do what is necessary. You are a mother goddess and you are powerful.

Take a deep breath and release some love to the Mother holding your feet. Wiggle your toes, releasing them. Spread your arms up overhead and bring your praying hands down to your heart center. Know you are loved and blessed. Bask in this love for a moment. When you are ready, open your eyes. Take a few minutes to rest before getting up from your comfortable position.

This meditation is a simple example of releasing and recharging, using the four elements. I made this up one day while in the bath and realized anyone can create their own meditation. Within each person, there is a sacred garden or quiet place that you can retreat to whenever needed. It all starts with visualizing your favorite escape. Whether it's the beach or a quiet trail in the mountains or sitting by a pool sipping a margarita, you can always go there and take a moment for yourself.

CHAPTER TEN

Accepting Help

As a new mother, you've probably heard, "When people offer to do your laundry or clean your floors, take them up on it." I'm here to say that's good advice. One of the biggest lessons I learned during my postpartum period was surrender of control. I didn't know I was such a control freak until I had my baby. Everything had to be a certain way and when things got out of hand, my mood did, too.

It wasn't long before I'd come to the realization that I couldn't do everything. It's practically impossible, especially if you've gone through a difficult labor or C-section. The body needs to recover and rest, all while caring for a new baby. Some things need to be delegated, like housework or cooking.

The first two weeks I was home, I kept people at a distance. I needed to recover from the trauma and face the realization I was now a mom. Withdrawing from the world led to isolation and loneliness. My friends and family offered to come over and take care of the housework or even hold my baby so I could do what I needed done, but I'd thank them for their offer and decline. A couple of my girlfriends ignored my polite refusals and came over anyway. Those precious hours they held Baby or switched out the laundry opened my eyes to the fact I needed help.

My own mother offered to cook for me, anything I wanted, even though she was vegan. It took about a month before I started letting her cook for me. Boy, did her meals make a difference. Instead of trying to figure out what to eat, I could focus on cleaning, checking my email, paying bills, or whatever else I wanted.

But help with housework and cooking wasn't the only help I needed. After a month of being cooped up in the house with a screaming infant, I desperately craved adult interactions and conversations. I started to hang out with my friends again and go to my women's circle group. Social interactions helped me break away from the black fog that seemed to have taken up permanent residence in my brain. We'll talk more about this in the next chapter.

Pelvic PT became a huge factor in helping me recover, both physically and emotionally. Knowing that the damaged tissue would heal and I wouldn't experience pain when inserting a small tampon did wonders to my spirit. I also discovered what I thought was "pushing" was quite the opposite. No wonder I couldn't get the baby out, I was doing it wrong.

About the time I went back to work, I'd realized I needed more than just physical attention. I needed psychological help. I still worried that I wasn't producing enough milk for my baby, even though she was at perfect weight. Every day I felt like the worst mother in the world and that I sucked at this new role in my life, even though I'd managed to keep my daughter safe and healthy for the past six months. The stress of my job, plus managing the rest of my life, still kept me up at night, but now I worked and couldn't nap with my girl during the day.

I never wanted to be one of "those" people that turned to medication for help, but at this point, desperation took over. The last thing I wanted was to lose my wonderful, well-paying job which provided financial independence and allowed me to work from home because of the poor state of my mind.

Swallowing my pride, I finally called my OB and told her what was happening. She first prescribed Wellbutrin, but I had a bad reaction after taking it for a week. She then switched me to a low dose of Zoloft. The effects took a while to kick in.

One evening after about two weeks of taking the new medication, I put Baby to bed and then went into the kitchen. In one hour, I cleaned the kitchen, washed the dishes, and swept all the floors in the house. As I jumped in the shower, I realized this was the first time I had done so many tasks without feeling like I was competing in a marathon. The dark fog began shifting into grey and slowly dispersed.

Anti-depression medication is a controversial issue for many, but I am now a firm believer that it has its place. It's not a long-term solution, but sometimes you need something extra to get you through a few months or even the first couple of years. I learned to put aside my pride and not feel guilty. I even shared this with people when they asked me how I was doing. I told them the truth, how I was dealing with depression and that now I was on medication and feeling better.

There's such a negative stigma around postpartum depression (PPD) and getting medical treatment for it. If you tell people you have diabetes or some other physical disease, it's no big deal, but the moment you mention depression or anything related to the mind, suddenly it is taboo and they look at you like you're crazy. I was lucky to have understanding friends and family, who were super supportive, but even then I've gotten the raised eyebrow every so often.

Postpartum depression is much more common than people realize. It's the one thing I didn't expect to deal with after childbirth. That's why I started writing this book. There needs to be more examples out there in terms of personal experience dealing with PPD and what helped women get through it. Postpartum depression is a real thing. I had a mild case of it compared to some mothers, but it doesn't matter the level of severity. PPD can affect anyone and can throw one's life into utter chaos.

Letting someone else do my laundry, clean my floor, buy groceries, wash the dishes, and take the garbage out became an exercise in releasing control and focusing on taking better care of myself so I could be there for my daughter. Getting help didn't mean I had failed as a mother.

Shortly after my daughter's first birthday, I finally bit another bullet and found a good therapist who specialized in women's mental health. She also was a mom and understood many of the things I was going through.

I cannot stress enough how important it is to have a trusted therapist who can help you. It's never too late to start. After talking to her at the first appointment, I discovered that I wasn't out of the danger zone. All of the tools that had helped thus far needed to be part of my everyday routine in order for me to continue down the path of recovery and health.

The most important thing I learned in the first year postpartum is that it really does take a village to raise a child and I had to let the village help me.

CHAPTER ELEVEN

Beautiful Relationships

Because it takes a village to raise a child, relationships are vital. I learned this important lesson the hard way. My natural attitude toward anything challenging is "do it my own way." Due to early life experiences, I became jaded about accepting others' help because it always came with strings attached. I had many friends, but that was because I put myself out there. As I got older and eventually found my mate, many of those relationships faded, but I still had many circles of friends.

When my daughter was born, I realized who my closest friends were. Those that kept their distance, I didn't blame. I had new priorities in my life besides going out for drinks or doing whatever singles or childless people do. However, having a diverse group of friendship proved to be a good thing. Each person contributed to my recovery in a unique way.

I also found new relationships forming. People I hadn't spoken with in years suddenly came to the surface because now they were mothers, too. Gals I hadn't hung out with much since they had children now became close friends again. I had a couple of friends who had babies around the same age as my daughter but most had girls or boys were a little older. I found the relationships with mothers of older children had the most value because they provided so much support and resources for a new mom like me. It was awesome being able to call them up and ask questions about something I didn't know. Plus, now we were in the same club. The motherhood club.

At the beginning of my pregnancy, my midwife gave me information for a mothers' group for women having their babies around the same time as me. At the time, I was working forty hours a week and we were planning on remodeling our home before the baby came. The thought of having to socialize after working long hours while being pregnant did not appeal to me. After I had my daughter, the midwife again strongly suggested I join the group but once again I didn't. This time depression and exhaustion were the excuses. The small amount of energy I had needed to be given to raising my new baby. Plus, I'm a natural introvert. Going out and meeting new people, even if they were moms, sounded like the worst assignment ever and I didn't want to be the Debbie-downer in the group.

Months later, however, I realized my mistake. Many of my mama friends had their mommy group pals who they did stuff with regularly. I wished I had some of those relationships, especially as my daughter got older and wanted to play.

In the fall, when Baby was eight months old, my Goddess Circle Sisters hosted a Fall Equinox retreat near Mt. Hood— six fabulous women plus offspring for a weekend of frivolous recreation and relaxation. At first, I thought it would be to a fantastic weekend, but as the time drew near, I started to panic and worry like there was no tomorrow.

What if my baby cried all night and kept everyone up? What if I was so tired I ended up being a lump on a log the entire time or a zombie mother staggering through the mountain cabin after my child? Worst of all, what if they confirmed I really was the worst mother in Earth's history?

In the end, all my worry was needless. The older kids watched over the little ones, which allowed us moms to have some good quality girl-time. My daughter made friends with the other kids, but she was the youngest. Watching her interact with the other kids made me wish I'd joined a mothers group with children similar in age to her.

But all was not lost. I discovered many activities in my town geared towards babies and toddlers. Our local library had story time for babies every week. I had a couple of girlfriends with infants around my daughter's age so I made a point to meet with these fine women at least once a month so my little one could interact with others on her level. The mamas got to have girl time, as well. It was a win-win situation.

In early October, I finally broke down and put my daughter in a Montessori daycare for a couple of days a week. She needed social interaction as much as I did, but I couldn't give it to her during the hours I had to work. This opened up more opportunities to interact with other mothers. My daughter's primary caregiver was a mom herself, and she offered me many amazing tips and solutions.

I finally joined a mothers' postpartum depression group through Baby Blues Connection more than a year after my daughter's birth. I wish I hadn't waited so long. Mothers need to stick together, and it's nice to know you're not alone in the trenches.

I know not everyone lives in a large city full of resources. Some live in the country or in rural areas. For those of you in that category, look online for mom groups. There are many parenting forums on the internet. Do your research and choose one that fits with your values and needs.

Reach out and build those bonds. They are invaluable to your sanity and will enrich your journey through motherhood-land.

Building relationships includes the one you have with your partner. Hubby and I have a wonderful marriage. We never fight and when we did have challenging times, we managed to get through, our bond becoming stronger each time.

Parenting, however, did take a huge toll on us. Luckily, we had a solid foundation under our marriage so when the storm clouds gathered, we were able to weather the tempest, but not without some scars.

Intimacy paid the greatest price. For the first three months postpartum, my soul craved it but my body and mind rejected any form whatsoever. I went through the motions of hugging and kissing my husband because I wanted him to know I loved him, but I felt nothing inside. Usually when he touched me he awakened every cell of my body, but I was dead inside. Cold as ice. This death started months before during my pregnancy.

Halfway through the second trimester, I stopped having orgasms during sex. I attributed this to my body changing with pregnancy and didn't worry about it too much. I was surprised I wasn't more aroused, as I'd heard countless women say the best sex they'd had was while pregnant. Maybe there was something wrong with me. I was wired differently, I guess.

After the trauma I had experienced to my genital area during childbirth, sex became the last thing on my mind. It scared the daylights out of me. Postpartum depression didn't help. I felt bad for my husband who patiently waited for me to make the first move. When I got the IUD, I thought maybe this was the beginning of my recovery and I'd be open to sex eventually.

The surgery that occurred a week later after the IUD insertion wiped that thought clean. I was so scared of the pain. I couldn't even touch myself down there without wincing. It was about a month after surgery that I attempted to pleasure myself, just to see if I still had the spark in me. It took almost an entire hour before anything happened. How depressing was that?

This only added to my growing lack of self-esteem. That's when I remembered the referral my OB had given me for pelvic PT. I started therapy. It was weird at first, as part of the treatment was inserting a finger into my vagina and stretching the tissue and massaging the scarred area. At one point my pelvic physical therapist suggested the use of a vibrator to ease my discomfort.

I started making an effort to cuddle with my husband for at least a couple of minutes a day, whether I felt like it or not. He loved being able to hold me because it made him feel like he was doing something with me again. Knowing this slowly melted the ice that had built around the cells of my body.

I made it a point to spend time together every week. Sometimes it was in the middle of the night when he woke up on his nights off from work. We'd eat a small meal together or I would take a bath so I could go back to sleep and he would hang out with me in the bathroom and chat. These moments fortified our relationship. I knew he loved me, and I was safe no matter what happened.

After months of therapy, I was I finally was able to have sex again. I remember the first time. Eight and half months after I had given birth, I made out with my husband and I realized that I was actually getting turned on. Eleven months postpartum, I started enjoying it and actually had an orgasm. That was the biggest breakthrough for me because I felt like a real woman once again.

Strengthening my relationships with my husband and friends helped me fight depression in so many ways.

CHAPTER TWELVE

Sacred Space

This, by far, was the hardest chapter to write for many reasons. I own a lot of stuff and my home is quite cluttered. It always amazed me how I would clean off the kitchen table and counters and a day later they were piled with papers, used bibs, dirty dishes, toys, electronics, keys, and who knows what else. Funny, how stuff seemed to appear out of thin air.

I would go through my closet and take several bags of stuff to Goodwill, only to have somebody give me just as many bags of baby stuff or items I'd ordered online would arrive. That's how fast the space I'd just cleared would fill back up.

My intentions of living in a clutter-free environment were good but not enough to make a difference. The more stuff that piled up on my desk, kitchen table, counter, and any other flat surface that wasn't the floor, the higher my stress level would rise.

Sometimes I would blame Hubby for not keeping things clean and organized, but truth be told, we were equally responsible for the clutter. He owns a lot of stuff, but I felt like a hypocrite, holding him accountable when my own desk and closet overflowed at critical mass.

When I read *The Art of Extreme Self Care* by Cheryl Richardson, I realized I had a serious problem. I bought too many things, and I held on to stuff far too long. When the house became a hoarder's wet dream, I became angry. Add postpartum depression to the mix and that's a delicious recipe for an explosive meltdown. Many months after I read the book and lots of soul-searching, I finally came to terms as to why my home looked more like a storage unit then a living space.

Fear. I held on to things because I was afraid I might need that item sometime. I kept many of the clothes my daughter had outgrown because I might get pregnant again. I kept receipts because I might need them to prove something someday. I bought stuff on sale, because, hello, you never should pass a good deal. And so on and so forth. Fear of not having enough was the root of the problem. My house filled up with junk, and I struggled to keep my credit card balance down, yet I still didn't have what I needed.

What brought this situation to the level of absurdity was the fact that I prided myself on being a minimalist. The outsider who never saw my home would think I lived by my mantra of simplicity. For example, when I go out with my daughter to run errands, I'm good for several hours with just a couple of diapers, a small travel pack of wipes, a pacifier, one small toy, a package of teething crackers, and a small cotton receiving blanket I keep in my purse. You don't need to haul around a huge diaper bag just to run to the store and grab some milk.

Yet my home looked like a hoarder's paradise. This had to end, especially since my mood tended to dip into the black side of things when the house was a mess. After much soul-searching, meditation, saging the house, and setting intentions, I started to declutter my home one drawer and closet at a time.

The process wasn't painless, but little by little, as I carried out bags of outgrown baby clothes and toys, I felt lighter and my brain felt less foggy. Craigslist and eBay became my friends as I sold many of my daughter's lightly used items and got some of my money back.

My home has always been a reflection of my mental state. When it's clean and organized, I feel great and everything seems to flow effortlessly. When it looks like a bomb has gone off, I can't focus on anything and bounce from one project to the next without actually finishing any of them. Frustration usually follows, with depression right on its heels, waving the "you suck" and "you can't do anything right" flags in my face.

Whenever I start down the spiral into the "suck vortex," I now look around the house and see what needs to be cleaned or put away. I force myself to get off my self-pity party ass and get to work. Some days though, energy and motivation are nowhere to be found. That's when I've learned to ask for help. Whether it is my mother taking her granddaughter for the day so I can have a breather or asking my husband to take the garbage out, seeking help doesn't come easy. But I've learned that my family and friends really do want to help; they just don't know how or when unless I let them know.

Once I have some alone time to think, breath, and rest, the energy and motivation show up and it's time to get stuff done.

But it's not just stuff in the home. I found that opening the blinds and windows to let sunshine and fresh air in can do miracles to the energy of the house.

Creating an environment that is nurturing, peaceful, and calm helps when dealing with postpartum depression or anxiety. And it can be done. Here are a few tips I've collected in my struggle with keeping a cleaner home:

Keep it simple. You don't need every gadget invented for moms and babies to survive. Discover what works for you and get rid of the excess.

Baby steps. Trying to declutter the entire nursery or closet in one fell swoop can be a daunting task. Start small—like one drawer or one corner of the closet each day. By the end of the week, you'll have the whole room transformed. Don't expect your house to be done in the snap of a finger. My first baby step was making sure my sink was free of dishes every night before bed. Supporting one clutter-free area spilled into cleaning off the counters on one side of the kitchen and then reorganizing my desk once a week.

Let go of the fear of having less. I had to ask myself, "What would my life be without this particular object?" If I found that it is necessary and I used it often, than it stayed. If it only took up space and I didn't need it, I considered letting it go. Imagine having fewer things to wash, put away, and organize. For every person this looks different. Find out what works for you and work toward that goal.

When you buy something new, get rid of something old. This is easiest when it comes to baby clothes since children grow so fast. I actually set a schedule on my phone calendar to clean out my daughter's dresser every three months and get rid of her out grown clothes, replacing them with the next size up of hand-me-downs and outfits I received as gifts.

Practice putting things away. It's so easy to come home and just drop everything on the chair by the door, but if you take time to hang up your coat, sort through the mail, etc., you will find that you have less stuff to clean or put away. It can be done. If you get in the habit of just doing one of the above, it makes a world of difference.

Keep baby toys to a minimum. Studies have shown that the fewer toys a child has in the first few years, the better creative skills they will develop through the use of their imagination. That doesn't mean you should deprive your child of toys but instead of piling all of their toys into one bin, get a couple of smaller boxes and put a few of toys in each. We did this with our daughter, and it turned out she played longer with one toy before moving on to the next when there was less. We also put toys in different parts of the house to encourage her to explore her environment and there was less for me to pick up at the end of the day.

You don't have to keep every gift you receive. People love to buy stuff for babies or pass on their children's outgrown clothing, but that doesn't mean you need to keep everything. While I was pregnant, I received dozens of bags of baby clothes from newborn to toddler sizes. At first I kept it all because I didn't know how fast my baby would grow and what size she'd reach during each season. After the first six months, I figured her trend and started sending bags to Goodwill. It felt good to make room after my closet had been packed full of baby clothes for months. What doesn't work for you doesn't need to stay, and there is no shame in that.

Decorate your home with things that make you happy. Whether you buy a vase of fresh flowers or place a candle on the counter or a green plant in the corner, fill your space with things that please you. For some, this may mean art or photos.

For others, mirrors or bright colors of paint. Whatever the object may be, make sure it inspires joy.

I had to remember to be kind to myself and not be too hard on myself if the process was slower than I would have liked or when results didn't meet my expectations. I knew I would get there eventually and soon be able to enjoy a home that made me smile and feel at ease. My house isn't perfect and I'm okay with it.

The Journey

Motherhood is a journey. While writing this book, I often asked myself what gave me the right to write a book about postpartum depression and how to get your life back after childbirth. Self-doubt always loves to mess with us, doesn't it?

Well, the answer to that is I've gone through this. Many people helped me out on my path to motherhood, and I wanted to pass along some of the lessons I'd learned to help other new moms make their lives better.

During the weeks around my daughter's first birthday, the flu bugs hit our home. First my husband, then me, and lastly my daughter. We passed two different bugs back and forth. I couldn't take my girl to daycare and my parents couldn't take her because my ten-month old nephew was staying with them for a couple of weeks. I didn't want him to get sick too. On top of no childcare, I had to work because I had some time-sensitive projects that needed to be done. In the course of two weeks, I remembered why I got so depressed.

No help, sleepless nights, stressful days, and a demanding baby led me back to square one. Luckily, I was working on revisions for this book at the same time and I remembered how I got out of darkness, too.

Depression is like a roller coaster. Just when you think you've cleared the woods suddenly there is a bend in the road and you find yourself plunging deeper into the darkness of the forest. I've learned to ride the waves as they come. Some days are easy; others feel like a marathon climb to the top of Everest.

It is my strong belief every mom can reclaim herself and live the life she desires while still being the mother she needs to be for her children. Being a new mom is hard, even if everything goes exactly how you want it to from the beginning. I learned to take one day at a time and be good to myself. I'm doing the best I can with what I have, like millions of other mothers around the world. I learned to ask for help and not to be afraid to say no to others' expectations or yes when people offer help. I learned I am beautiful. I am a mother. I am a queen. So I lift my chin, straighten my spine, and hold my head high. I might not be perfect but I still am the goddess of my home and life.

RESOURCES

Books

Slow-Down Therapy by Linus Munday and *New Baby Therpay* by Lisa O. Engelhardt, Elf-Help books, Abbey Press.

The Art of Extreme Self-Care by Cheryl Richardson, Hay House.

Down Came the Rain by Brook Shields, Hyperion.

The Mommy Myth: The Idealization of Motherhood and How It Has Undermined Women by Susan J. Douglas and Meredith Michaels, Simon and Schuster.

Yoga for Mother and Baby by Julie Llewellyn-Thomas, MITCH.

Simplify by Joshua Becker, available on Kindle.

Websites

www.chopracentermeditation.com
www.postpartum.net
www.rachaelray.com
www.kellymom.com

ACKNOWLEDGEMENTS

I want to thank my awesome beta-readers Vanessa, Laura, and Amy. To Maria Connor at My Author Concierge for helping hone my writing skills through editing. Your support and encouragement gave me the confidence to tell my story. To Kathleen McFall for your endless kindness and support in my writing endeavors and for cheering me on this project. To Christy Carlyle for the beautiful cover. To Delilah, Jessa and the rest of my friends at Rose City Romance Writers for encouraging me to share my story.

To all of my family and friends who loved me unconditionally and supported me through this journey. To my magical circle of Spiral Wise women who held me during my darkest moments these last couple of years. My soul sisters, Sarah and Melissa.

Many thanks to Dr. Robin Barrett for giving me hope in the midst of the storm.

To my dear husband, Eric, for being my safety harness through this crazy roller coaster ride. I couldn't have done it without you. I love you so much.

Last but not least to my sweet little princess, Elly. You have taught me so much from the day you were born. I love you to the end of the universe and back, baby. Because of you, I'm a much better person today. Thank you for choosing me to be your mommy.

ABOUT THE AUTHOR

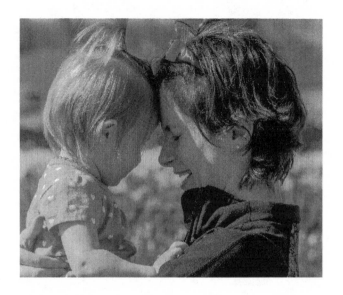

Melania can be found wearing comfy yoga pants in her
modest kitchen stirring a boiling pot of organic pasta, feeding
little Boo Creature fresh veggies, balancing a phone between
her shoulder and cheek, all the while petting one of her feline
beasts with a foot. She has been known to dance to an Irish
jig. You can also find her at
www.urbangoddessrevealed.blogspot.com.

Urban Goddess Mama-to-Be
Coming November 2014